# THE COMPLETE LOW CARB BOOK

## Quick and Delicious Recipes
## For Family and Friends
## incl. 2 Weeks LC Meal Prep Plan

MATTHEW BAILEY

ISBN- 9798519002516

# TABLE OF CONTENTS

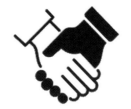

# Introduction

Losing weight, maintaining weight, and living a generally healthy lifestyle sound like they should be easy endeavours. In reality however, they're far from it!

There are so many fad diets out there, it's easy to become confused about what you should do versus what you shouldn't. Dedicating yourself to a healthier lifestyle doesn't have to be complicated. You don't have to restrict your intake of certain foods to the point of extreme cravings. Instead, you just need to arm yourself with the knowledge of what you need versus what you don't, whilst throwing in a good amount of moderation.

Have you heard of the low carb lifestyle?

Yes, when you're following a low carb diet you're lowering the amount of carbs you're consuming but not to the point where you're going to have raging cravings. If anything, after the first phase of the diet, you'll have far less cravings because you're eating wholesome and delicious foods, which are naturally more satiating.

Sounds good, right?

We're constantly bombarded with advice that knowing the right line to go down can be hard. Why not simplify it and give the low carb lifestyle a try?

All you need to do is less less carbs, more fat, a little more protein, and make sure you vary up your meals so you don't become bored. Then, once you see the results coming your way, you won't want to stop!

To simplify everything beyond measure, we've put together your go-to guide for everything low carb. From what you need to do versus what you don't, how to prepare your kitchen, and what the lifestyle actually involves, we cover it all. Then, we're going to give you some delicious and easy to create recipes for breakfasts, lunches, dinners, and even desserts. You'll be spoilt for choice!

Of course, getting started on any diet or lifestyle change is the hardest part. We're going to make that easy too, by outlining a 2 week-long meal prep guide. Mix up the meals if you want to, but you can easily see how to put together your meals throughout the week and hit your weight loss/maintenance or general health targets.

Optimum health doesn't have to be difficult and it certainly doesn't have to mean boring and uninspiring meals. If anything, it means the opposite!

So, without further ado, let's delve into the world of low carb and show you just how easy it can be.

# Low Carb Lifestyle – What's It All About?

Before you jump right into cooking low carb dishes, you need to understand the lifestyle you're about to embark upon. If you don't understand it, you'll end up eating the wrong things, doing the wrong things and it won't give you the results you're after.

The good news is that there isn't a huge amount of information to bear in mind, you just need to have a few hints and tips up your sleeve to keep you on the right track.

Before we get into the good stuff, i.e. the recipes, let's outline what the low carb diet is, what it isn't, and how to follow it effectively.

## How to Follow The Low Carb Lifestyle

You'll no doubt have heard of low carb before. The Keto Diet has been around for many years and this is one of the most famous low carb lifestyles around. However, the Keto Diet is a little stricter than a regular low carb diet needs to be. In fact, we won't call it a diet, because that's not really what it is.

If you're going to do low carb, you need to stick to it. You can't dip in and out of it because you're going to confuse your body. The reason is down to something called ketosis.

Let's have a quick biology lesson.

When you're following a regular eating plan, i.e. you're not reducing any particular food group and you're eating freely, your body burns the carbohydrates you consume for energy. This isn't just energy to go out and do your shopping etc, but energy for the things that your body needs to do in order to stay healthy and function effectively.

When you reduce the amount of carbs you're consuming, your brain suddenly notices the drop and starts to panic for a second. Where is the energy going to come from?! Because the brain is always looking for threats to your health, a basic way that it keeps you alive, it deems the lower amount of carbohydrates to burn for energy as a huge threat. It thinks it's going to starve.

Now in reality, you're not going to starve. To counteract the threat, your body pushes you into a new metabolic state, called ketosis. This is basically turning the fat burning switch on. Your body starts to produce ketones in the liver, which are derived from fat proteins. In order to keep producing these ketones and therefore have enough energy to burn for all the things your body needs, you have to eat more of the good types of fat.

Confused?

Bear with it!

You're eating more fat (to a certain amount and only healthy fats) which means your body has an energy source, but you're also eating into your fat stores. For that reason, you're likely to notice a good weight loss in the first week or two, before it slows down to a regular and manageable amount. Then, when you find your happy medium of how many carbohydrates you need to consume in order to feel good and stay at your current weight, you enter a maintenance phase that is ongoing.

To sum up briefly, when you lower the amount of carbs you eat, you turn the fat burning switch on. That helps you to get rid of any fat stores that are just sat there doing nothing currently, whilst burning the fats that you're eating.

It's so simple once you break it down!

The major worry with cutting down on any major food group is whether or not it is safe. As long as you make sure you're eating enough of the right kinds of fats (not the saturated or processed kinds), you're getting enough protein in your diet, and you're not dipping in and out of it by eating lots of carbs one day and then none the next few days, it's perfectly healthy for most people.

Of course, if you have any health concerns, especially diabetes, you should talk to your doctor before embarking on a low carb lifestyle. It may be that you need to adapt it to your needs, but that is something your doctor will be able to advise you on.

The first couple of weeks may bring cravings your way, but stick with it because once your body adjusts, it will be much easier from there on in. You'll then slowly find your carb happy level and you'll feel fanatic on the inside too.

You might be wondering how many carbs actually counts as 'low'. There are many low carb diets out there and they all have different guidelines, ranging between 20-50 grams per day. When looking for recipes to try or foods to purchase, opt for those which are low in carb intake, e.g. in the single figures, but higher in nutritional amount. You need to think about fresh fruits, fresh vegetables, lean meats, and whole, organic, and natural items.

Low carb doesn't only mean low carb however, it also means high fat and moderate protein. How much protein? That also varies. A good guideline is between 0.7 to 0.9g of protein per every pound of your body weight. Everyone is different and we all need slightly different amounts of protein.

Of course, when it comes to fat, we're talking about healthy fats, such as those found in fatty fish (omega 3 fatty acids), tofu, soy, walnuts, sunflower seeds, and coconut milk. In fact, coconut milk is a great choice for those who do enjoy milk (you'll find out why shortly) because they're high in MCTs, or medium-chain triglycerides - a type of healthy fat.

The main benefits of a low carb diet are:
- Less cravings
- Regulated appetite
- Weight loss
- May lead to lower cholesterol levels
- May lead to lower blood sugar levels and in some cases, may help with diabetes control
- May lower hypertension (blood pressure)
- More energy

## Foods to Eat, Foods to Avoid

When you start reading about low carb lifestyles, you'll automatically see the Ketogenic Diet, or the Keto Diet, crop up. That is a low carb option but it's a little stricter and more regimented than a simple low carb option. For that reason, no particular food is outlawed on a low carb lifestyle, but there are definitely foods that you should limit, usually foods which are naturally high in carbs.

Of course, you should also cut out processed foods and extremely unhealthy options, such as saturated fat. This is the same with any effort to live more healthily and lose weight.

In this section, let's look at the foods you should perhaps give a wide berth to, those you should limit, and those you can eat freely.

## Avoid, Avoid, Avoid!

- Bread or bread-related products, such as tortillas, bagels, etc – don't panic however, you can still make low carb bread if you really need it in your life!
- Cakes, chocolate, sweets, etc – we're going to show you how to make some delicious low carb desserts later on, so don't despair just yet
- Pasta. Again, you can make your own low carb version by using spiralised vegetables instead
- Cereals, including oatmeal, granola, and muesli
- Beer. If you really enjoy an alcoholic beverage from time to time, stick to wine or spirits instead
- Fruit juices – stick to the natural variety!
- Sugar, including natural sugars, such as honey or maple syrup

## Proceed With Caution

- Certain fruits that are naturally high in carbs, such as bananas, mangoes, raisins, and dates
- Certain starchy vegetables, such as corn, potatoes, sweet potatoes or yams, and beets
- Sweetened yogurt – stick to plain natural yogurt or Greek yogurt
- Salad dressings, including those which are advertised as being 'low fat' or even 'fat free' – they may be low in fat but they're not low in carbs, and remember, you need fat!
- Legumes - it's a good idea to consume some legumes, such as lentils,

peas, black beans, kidney beans, and chickpeas, but keep it to a moderate amount as these can easily take you towards high carb amounts

- Milk – a small amount of milk is fine, e.g. in your morning tea or coffee, but avoid drinking glasses of milk or adding too much to recipes

**Go Ahead, Knock Yourself Out!**

- Unsweetened dairy products
- Fish
- Eggs
- Lean meat and poultry
- Leafy greens
- Nuts and seeds
- Healthy oils, such as olive oil, rapeseed oil, and coconut oil
- Cauliflower
- Broccoli
- Certain fruits, including blueberries, strawberries, and apples in particular

## Preparing Your Kitchen For Low Carb Cooking

Before you start embarking upon your new low carb lifestyle, it's a good idea to lay a solid foundation. If your kitchen cupboards are full of bread, bagels, cakes, and cookies, you're going to find it hard to resist when you're in the first week or two of the new lifestyle and you're having the odd craving.

Evaluate one cupboard at a time and discard anything that doesn't fit in with your new healthy lifestyle. If it still has life left in it, gift it to someone else rather than throwing it away and adding to waste. Make sure you also go through your refrigerator and your freezer.

Then, when you're sure that you have nothing in there that doesn't fit in, it's time to go shopping and stock up on all the things you're going to need for your new cooking adventure. The great thing about going low carb is that you're going to be focusing on home cooking. By doing that, you're not only ensuring that you stick to your lifestyle but you're also going to appreciate the tastes, flavours and textures of your food so much more - you're the one making it!

The staple basics you'll need are:
- Olive oil
- Coconut oil
- Herbs and spices
- Salt and pepper
- Psyllium husk (used in place of flour)
- Powdered erythritol (a low carb sweetener)
- Eggs

That doesn't sound like much but these are the ingredients that you'll need in your cupboard that you'll use time and time again. The rest, such as fresh produce and meat, can be bought as you outline your weeks meal plan.

Speaking of meal plans, it's a great idea to sit down on a Sunday evening and work out your meals for the week. By doing that, you'll not only eliminate those "what shall we have for dinner" questions every single day, but you'll also save money because you have everything you need in the house.

Once you've created your meal plan, you'll go shopping and get everything you need. Of course, you can mix things up once or twice during the week if you're really not feeling what you've planned, but try to stick to your plan as much a possible and vary your meals as much as possible, to stop you from becoming bored and also to ensure that you get a good range of nutrition from your meals.

## The Do's And Don'ts of Low Carb Life

We're almost onto the good bit - the recipes! Before we head there however, let's quickly look at a few important do's and don'ts of the low carb lifestyle.

**Do's**

- **Drink plenty of water** – Hydration is important at any time but when you're on a low carb routine, this will help to flush out toxins quicker and ensure optimum health
- **Plan your meals ahead to save time and effort** – We've just talked about meal planning and it really will make such a difference to your day. It also puts you in control of your daily nutritional needs
- **Try new things and mix up your meals** – One of the main reasons people "fall off the diet wagon" is because their meals become too repetitive and boring. Mix things up and try new things – go on, be brave!

**Don'ts**

- **Skips meals** – Make sure you have three proper meals every day to ensure your blood sugar levels remain stable
- **Dip in and out of the low carb lifestyle** – You need to be on it or off it and nothing in-between. When your body goes into ketosis, it needs to stay there for as long as you're planning on sticking with low carb. If you dip in

and out, you're going to end up with side effects you may not find pleasant, such as headaches, stomach upsets, problems sleeping, tiredness, etc.

- **Assume you can't have a treat occasionally** – Moderation is key in any lifestyle. You need to have the things you enjoy but the key word is 'moderation'. If you have a snack that could be considered high in carbs, don't worry about it as long as you only have it once, very rarely. Life is too short to completely cut out your favourite foods!

So, now you know all the facts, are you ready to delve into some delicious low carb recipes?

# Breakfast Recipes

# SALMON, SPINACH & EGGS

*Servings - 1*
*Carbs - 2g, fat - 34g, protein - 25g, calories - 419*

## INGREDIENTS

- 1 tbsp butter
- 2 eggs
- 55g smoked salmon
- 2 tbsp double cream
- 28g spinach
- Salt and pepper for seasoning

## METHOD

1. Take a large frying pan and add the butter over a medium heat
2. Add the spinach and cook until soft
3. Pour the cream into the pan and cook until thick
4. Add the eggs and combine well
5. Season and cook until the eggs are to your liking
6. Serve the eggs on the plate with the salmon by the side

# ONION & BACON BREAKFAST PANCAKE

*Servings - 4*
*Carbs - 5g, fat - 49g, protein - 22g, calories - 553*

## INGREDIENTS

- 2 tbsp butter
- 100g bacon
- Half an onion
- 4 eggs
- 240ml double cream
- 120ml almond flour
- 120ml cottage cheese
- 1 tsp baking powder
- 1 tbsp psyllium husk powder
- Salt and pepper for seasoning

## METHOD

1. Preheat the oven to 175C
2. Cut the bacon into small pieces, along with the onion
3. Take a frying pan and add the butter, over a medium heat
4. Cook the bacon and the onion is soft and the bacon is crispy
5. Take a mixing bowl and add the cream, cottage cheese and the eggs, combining well
6. Add the flour, psyllium husk, baking powder and a little salt
7. Combine well and place to one side for a while
8. Take a baking tray and grease well
9. Pour the batter onto the tray and move around to spread
10. Add the bacon and onion on top of the batter
11. Place in the oven for 20 minutes and cook until browned and set in the middle
12. Cut into pieces and serve

# TURKEY & MUSTARD BREAKFAST SANDWICH

*Servings - 4*
*Carbs - 5g, fat - 17g, protein - 10g, calories - 212*

## INGREDIENTS

- 4 tbsp mayonnaise
- 110g sliced turkey (deli meat)
- 4 large pickles
- 0.5 tbsp Dijon mustard
- 1 sliced tomato
- 2 lettuce leaves
- Quarter sliced red onion
- 55g sliced cheddar cheese

## METHOD

1. Take the pickles and slice lengthways, removing the seeds and creating a boat shape
2. Take a mixing bowl and combine the mustard and the mayonnaise
3. Add the mixture to the inside of the pickles
4. Add the turkey, lettuce, tomato, red onion, and finally the cheese
5. Take the other pickle and place on top, like a bread bun
6. Use a toothpick to hold the "sandwich" together

# MACKEREL & EGGS

*Servings - 2*
*Carbs - 4g, fat - 59g, protein - 35g, calories - 689*

## INGREDIENTS

- 2 tbsp butter
- 60ml olive oil
- 4 eggs
- 1 can of mackerel in tomato sauce
- Half a red onion, sliced
- 60g lettuce
- Salt and pepper for seasoning

## METHOD

1. Take a frying pan and add the butter over a medium heat
2. Add the eggs to the pan and cook them to your liking
3. Take a serving plate and add the lettuce down first then the slices of red onion, and the mackerel
4. Serve the eggs on top
5. Season to your liking and add the olive oil over the top in a drizzle

# BACON & AVOCADO EGGS

*Servings - 2*
*Carbs - 2g, fat - 31g, protein - 25g, calories - 407*

## INGREDIENTS

- 1 tsp olive oil
- 4 eggs
- 70g bacon
- Half an avocado, peeled and stone removed
- Salt and pepper for seasoning

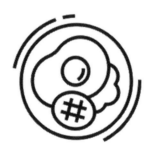

# METHOD

1. Preheat your oven to 180C
2. Take a baking tray and line with baking parchment
3. Place the bacon on the tray and leave to rest to one side
4. Take a saucepan and fill with cold water, leaving 2cm over the top of the eggs when you add them inside
5. Cover the pan and cook over a high heat
6. Once the water is boiling rigorously, remove the pan and place to one side, allowing to rest for 15 minutes
7. Take a large spoon and remove the eggs from the pan and place in a bowl of cold water for up to 10 minutes
8. Remove the shells and place the eggs to one side
9. Place the bacon in the oven and cook for 15 minutes, until crispy
10. Remove the bacon and place on paper towel, to absorb the oil
11. Once the bacon is cool, cut into triangles
12. Cut the eggs in half lengthways and use a spoon to remove the yolks
13. Take a mixing bowl and add the yolks with the olive oil and the avocado
14. Use a fork to mash the mixture together until smooth
15. Season to your liking and combine once more
16. Spoon the mixture into the eggs and top with a piece of the bacon
17. Season and serve

# AVOCADO & SWEDE FRITTERS

*Servings - 4*
*Carbs - 12g, fat - 66g, protein - 23g, calories - 756*

## INGREDIENTS

### For the fritters:

- 3 tbsp coconut flour
- 55g butter
- 230g halloumi cheese
- 4 eggs
- 450g swede
- A pinch of turmeric
- Salt and pepper for seasoning

### Mayonnaise mixture & serving:

- 1 tbsp ranch seasoning
- 120ml mayonnaise
- 2 avocados, peeled and stone removed, sliced
- 140g leafy greens

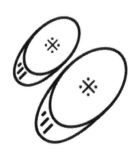

# METHOD

1. Preheat your oven to 120C
2. Peel the swede and grate coarsely
3. Shred the cheese
4. Take a mixing bowl and add the cheese, eggs, swede, coconut flour, seasoning and turmeric, combining well
5. Sit for 5 minutes to rest
6. Take a large frying pan and add the butter over a medium heat
7. Use your hands to form three patties with the mixture, around 0.5cm thickness
8. Cook the patties for 4 minutes on each side
9. Take a mixing bowl and combine the mayonnaise and ranch to create a sauce
10. Serve the fritters with the mayonnaise mixture on top
11. Arrange the leafy greens and sliced avocado at the side

# MORNING CAPRESE OMELETTE

*Servings - 2*
*Carbs - 4g, fat - 42g, protein - 42g, calories - 533*

## INGREDIENTS

- 2 tbsp olive oil
- 140g sliced fresh mozzarella cheese
- 6 eggs
- 1 tbsp fresh basil, chopped
- 85g halved cherry tomatoes
- Salt and pepper for seasoning

## METHOD

1. Take a mixing bowl and crack the eggs inside, seasoning to your liking
2. Use a fork to whisk and combine the eggs
3. Add the chopped basil and combine again
4. Take a frying pan and add the oil over a medium heat
5. Cook the tomatoes for a minute or two on both sides
6. Pour the egg over the tomatoes and move the pan to spread the mixture around
7. When the omelette has started to firm a little, add the mozzarella and cook for a few extra minutes
8. Serve whilst hot

# BREAKFAST TACO TURNOVER

*Servings - 2*
*Carbs - 8g, fat - 63g, protein - 44g, calories - 790*

## INGREDIENTS

### For the turnover:

- 140g ground beef
- 1 tbsp olive oil
- 4 eggs
- 1 avocado
- 140g grated cheddar cheese
- The juice of 1 lime
- 1 diced tomato
- 1 tsp fresh coriander
- Salt and pepper for seasoning

### For the taco mixture:

- 0.5 tsp cumin, ground
- 0.25 tsp onion powder
- 0.5 tsp paprika
- 0.5 tsp garlic powder
- 0.5 tsp fresh oregano (dried would also work well)
- 0.25 tsp chilli flakes
- 0.5 tsp salt
- 0.25 tsp black pepper

# METHOD

1. Take a small bowl and combine all the spices for the taco mixture, mixing well
2. Take a large frying pan and add the ground beef
3. Add the taco mixture and stir well, to ensure the ground beef is totally combined
4. Fry over a medium heat until the meat is cooked
5. Remove the pan from the heat and remove the meat, placing to one side
6. Take a mixing bowl and add the eggs, whisking until combined
7. Turn the heat down and take the same frying pan you used earlier
8. Add the eggs and cook until the edges start to firm up
9. Use a spatula to ease the edges and move the uncooked egg to the middle
10. Cook for a couple of minutes, until firming up
11. Add the lime juice to the cooked beef and combine
12. Take the avocado and cut it in half, removing the stone and scooping out the middle
13. Cut the avocado flesh into pieces
14. Add the beef on top of the omelette and top with three quarter of the cheese
15. Add the tomatoes as a final topping
16. Carefully remove the omelette from the frying pan and fold
17. Add the rest of the cheese on top, the avocado, and the cilantro, with a little seasoning
18. Serve whilst still hot

# BERRY BREAKFAST SMOOTHIE

*Servings - 2*
*Carbs - 10g, fat - 42g, protein - 4g, calories - 416*

## INGREDIENTS

- 140g sliced fresh strawberries
- 1 tbsp lime juice
- 425ml coconut milk
- 0.5 tsp vanilla extract

## METHOD

1. Take a blender and add all ingredients inside
2. Blend until everything is smooth
3. Add a little extra lime juice if you like a zinger taste
4. Serve immediately

# AVOCADO EGGS BENEDICT

*Servings - 4*
*Carbs - 3g, fat - 47g, protein - 17g, calories - 516*

## INGREDIENTS

- 4 eggs
- 3 extra egg yolks
- 110g butter
- 1 tbsp fresh lemon juice
- 2 avocados, skin and stone removed
- 140g smoked salmon
- Salt and pepper for seasoning

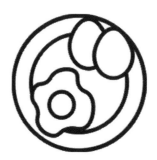

# METHOD

1. Melt the butter either over a low heat in a saucepan or in the microwave
2. Add the melted butter to a mixing bowl and add the yolks and the lemon juice
3. Use an immersion blender to combine until creamy
4. Add salt and pepper and combine again
5. Take a saucepan and add some water, bringing to the boil
6. Take a measuring cup and crack the eggs inside individually
7. As you crack one egg, slide one egg into the water at a time, cooking for 4 minutes to poach
8. Use a slotted spoon to remove the eggs from the water and place on a paper towel
9. Take the avocados and cut a slice off the bottom so they will stand up on a plate
10. Add one egg to one half of avocado and a spoonful of the sauce on top
11. Add a little smoked salmon at the side
12. Eat immediately

# Lunch Recipes

# MINI HAM QUICHES

*Servings - 4*
*Carbs - 4g, fat - 37g, protein - 32g, calories - 490*

## INGREDIENTS

- 8 eggs
- 400g sliced ham
- 200g cream cheese
- 3 tbsp chopped chives (fresh work best)
- Salt and pepper for seasoning

## METHOD

1. Preheat your oven to 180C
2. Take 4 ramekins which are suitable for the oven and grease with a little butter or oil
3. Take a piece of ham and place in the bottom of each ramekin, creating a crust by covering the sides and the bottom
4. Take a mixing bowl and add the cream cheese, eggs, chives, and a little seasoning, whisking together until smooth
5. Distribute the mixture equally between each ramekin and place in the oven for 15 minutes
6. Eat whilst still warm

# SHRIMP & CABBAGE STIR FRY

*Servings - 2*
*Carbs - 12g, fat - 20g, protein - 38g, calories - 389*

## INGREDIENTS

- 2 tbsp coconut oil
- 300g shrimps, defined and peeled
- 2 finely chopped garlic cloves
- 450g sliced cabbage
- 2 tbsp soy sauce
- 2 tbsp chopped fresh ginger
- The juice of 1 lime
- 2 tbsp sesame seeds
- 8g fresh, chopped coriander
- Salt and pepper for seasoning

## METHOD

1. Take a large frying pan and add half of the oil over a medium heat
2. Add the garlic, ginger, and cabbage, cooking for a minute, before strong
3. Cook until the cabbage is soft
4. Add the soy sauce, coriander, lime juice and sesame seeds and combine again
5. Take another pan and cook the shrimp in the rest of the oil, cook for around 6 minutes
6. Arrange the cabbage mixture on the plates and add the shrimp on top of t
7. Use a spoon to distribute the juices from the pan over the top and add a few extra sesame seeds as a garnish

# FETA TABBOULEH BOWL

*Servings - 2*
*Carbs -11g, fat - 50g, protein - 28g, calories - 621*

## INGREDIENTS

- 2 tbsp olive oil
- 70g feta cheese
- 85g prosciutto
- 100g cauliflower florets
- 14g chopped spring onions
- Half a diced tomato
- 2 tsp lemon juice
- 60ml fresh mint
- Salt and pepper for seasoning

## METHOD

1. Take a large salad bowl and add the small cauliflower florets, tomato, lemon juice, spring onions, tomato, lemon juice and the mint, seasoning and combining together
2. Mix well and leave aside for 20 minutes
3. Break the feta into small pieces and arrange over the top of the bowl
4. Shred the prosciutto and sprinkle over the top

# LOW CARB TUNA BURGERS

*Servings - 4*
*Carbs - 8g, fat - 58g, protein - 39g, calories - 722*

## INGREDIENTS

- 3 tbsp olive oil
- 1 can of tuna, drained
- 2 eggs
- 180ml mayonnaise, plus an extra 4 tbsp for serving
- 2 tbsp onion powder
- 2 tbsp garlic powder
- 2 sliced tomatoes
- 85g lettuce
- Salt and pepper for seasoning

## METHOD

1. Take a large mixing bowl and combine the tuna, 180ml mayonnaise, garlic powder, onion powder, eggs, and seasoning
2. Use your hands to form patties with the mixture; you should be able to create 4 large patties
3. Take a large frying pan and add the oil over a medium heat
4. Cook for 3-4 minutes on each side, until crispy
5. Add some lettuce to your serving plates and add a tuna burger on top
6. Add a slice of tomato on top of the burger and a spoonful of the mayonnaise for serving
7. Season and enjoy

# MOZZARELLA BEEF SALAD

*Servings - 6*
*Carbs - 3g, fat - 65g, protein - 43g, calories - 784*

## INGREDIENTS

- 2 tbsp olive oil
- 1 minced garlic clove
- 900g sirloin steak
- 300g cherry tomatoes, cut into halves
- 160g leafy greens
- 300g mozzarella balls
- 1 tbsp fresh basil
- 0.5 tbsp oregano
- 2 tbsp fresh parsley
- 3 tbsp cider vinegar
- 180ml extra virgin olive oil
- 2 tbsp Dijon mustard
- Salt and pepper for seasoning

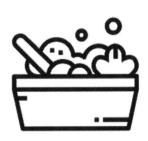

# METHOD

1. Take a large frying pan and allow to reach a medium to high temperature
2. Take the steak and season with little salt and pepper
3. Take a mixing bowl and add the 2 tbsp olive oil and garlic, coming well
4. Brush the mixture over both sides of the steak
5. Place the steak into the frying pan and cook for 4 minutes on both sides
6. Remove the steak from the pan and place to one side with a little foil over the top, leave to sit for around 5 minutes
7. Take a large salad bowl and add the leafy greens and cherry tomatoes inside, along with the mozzarella, combining well
8. Take a blender and add the basil, oregano, parsley, extra virgin olive oil, cider vinegar, Dijon mustard and a little seasoning, combining well with the blender
9. Slice the beef thinly and add into the salad bowl, combining carefully
10. Drizzle the dressing over the top and season to your liking

# LEEK & BROCCOLI SOUP WITH CHEESY CHIPS

*Servings - 4*
*Carbs - 12g, fat - 53g, protein - 17g, calories - 590*

## INGREDIENTS

- 700ml vegetable stock
- 1 leek
- 280g broccoli
- 200g cream cheese
- 240ml double cream
- 21g chopped fresh basil
- 1 pressed garlic clove
- 350ml grated cheddar cheese
- 0.5 tsp paprika
- Salt and pepper for seasoning

# METHOD

1. Take the leek and wash well, removing the outer parts. Slice the rest into the slices and allow to sit in a bowl of cold water
2. After a few minutes, drain the water and pat the leeks dry
3. Slice the broccoli into the slices and place to one side
4. Take a large soup pot and add the leek and broccoli
5. Add the stock and cover the pot, bringing to the boil
6. Cook until the broccoli is soft
7. Add the cream cheese, double cream and the rest of the ingredients, except for the cheddar and paprika
8. Blend the soup with an immersion blender until smooth
9. Preheat the oven to 200C
10. Take a large baking tray and line with parchment paper
11. Add the cheese to the baking tray in medium sized mounds and make sure there is enough space in-between
12. Add a little paprika on top and bake in the oven for 5 minutes
13. Serve with the soup

# TRADITIONAL GUMBALAYA

*Servings - 10*
*Carbs - 8g, fat - 22g, protein - 36g, calories - 392*

## INGREDIENTS

- 120ml coconut oil
- 2 minced garlic cloves
- 1kg chicken thighs, no bones, cut into cubes
- 450g shrimp, deveined and peeled
- 350g sliced spicy sausage, any you like
- 3 chopped celery stalks
- 1 onion
- 1 green bell pepper
- 2 cans of crushed tomatoes
- 120ml water
- 475ml beef broth
- 85g okra
- 1 tsp cajun powder
- 1 tsp gumbo file powder
- 0.5 tsp cayenne pepper
- 1 tsp salt

# METHOD

1. Take a large frying pan and add the coconut oil over a medium heat
2. Add chicken and the garlic and cook until the chicken is browned
3. Slice the onion and pepper and add to the pan, combining well
4. Add the cayenne, cajun and the gumbo file, combining well
5. Add the salt and combine again, cooking for another minute
6. Add the spicy sausage, tomatoes, okra, celery, broth, and water, combining well
7. Allow the pan to boil lightly, until it starts to become thicker
8. Turn the heat down a little and allow to simmer for 15 minutes
9. Add the shrimp and continue simmering for around 3 minutes, until the shrimp is cooked
10. Serve!

# CAULIFLOWER & MUSHROOM RISOTTO

*Servings - 2*
*Carbs - 13g, fat - 48g, protein - 12g, calories - 557*

## INGREDIENTS

- 110g butter
- 1 cauliflower (around 850g in weight)
- 260g mushrooms
- 240ml vegetable stock
- 240ml double cream
- 2 cloves of garlic
- 1 spring onion, chopped finely
- 180ml white wine
- 40g grated parmesan cheese
- Salt and pepper for seasoning

## METHOD

1. Take a large frying pan and add the butter over a medium heat
2. Cook the mushrooms until they're a golden brown colour
3. Add the spring onion and the garlic and combine
4. Grate the cauliflower and add to the frying pan, combining again
5. Add the stock and half of the wine, stirring well
6. Leave the lid off and allow the mixture to simmer until it starts to reduce
7. Add the rest of the wine, cream, and continue to simmer until most of the liquid has gone
8. Remove the pan from the heat and add the cheese, stirring well

# TACO FISH BOWL

*Servings - 2*
*Carbs - 12g, fat - 61g, protein - 38g, calories - 769*

## INGREDIENTS

- 2 tbsp olive oil
- 220g green or red cabbage, depending upon your preference
- 1 tomato
- Half an onion
- 1 avocado
- 1 tbsp Tex-Mex seasoning (fajita would also work)
- 325g any white fish of your choice
- 60ml mayonnaise
- 1 tbsp lime juice
- 0.5 tsp garlic powder
- 1 tsp hot sauce
- Salt and pepper for seasoning

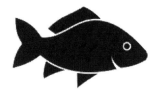

# METHOD

1. Create your dressing first and allow to marinade - take a large mixing bowl and add the lime juice, hot sauce, garlic powder, and the mayonnaise, combining well. Season to your liking and place to one side

2. Shred the tomato, onion and cabbage into thin slices with a very sharp knife

3. Take the avocado and cut in half, removing the stone

4. Remove the flesh with a spoon and slice

5. Arrange all the vegetables onto a serving plate and season

6. Drizzle the oil over the top and place to one side

7. Take a large frying pan and add a little oil, over a medium heat

8. Add a little salt to both sides of the fish and place in the pan, cooking for 3 minutes on each side

9. Once cooked, cut the fish into smaller pieces and arrange on the serving plate

10. Pour the dressing over the top and combine well before serving

# CREAM CHEESE PANCAKES

*Servings - 4*
*Carbs - 7g, fat - 38g, protein - 18g, calories - 447*

## INGREDIENTS

### For the pancakes:

- 260g cottage cheese
- 5 eggs
- 1 tbsp psyllium husk
- A pinch of salt
- A little butter for frying

### For the cream cheese topping:

- 2 tbsp green pesto
- 230g cream cheese
- 2 tbsp olive oil
- Half a sliced red onion
- Salt and pepper for seasoning

## METHOD

1. Take a medium bowl and add the pesto, cream cheese, and 1 tbsp olive oil, combining well and leaving to one side

2. Take 2 tbsp of butter and add to a frying pan, over a medium heat

3. Use two spoons of the cottage cheese to create a pancake shape in the pan, around 3 inches wide

4. Cook for 2 minutes and turn, cooking for the same amount of time on the other side

5. Pile the pancakes on your plate and serve with the cream cheese dressing

6. Top with the red onion and season with a drizzle of oil over the top

# Dinner Recipes

# CAULIFLOWER GRATIN & PORK CHOPS

*Servings - 6*
*Carbs - 9g, fat - 56g, protein - 41g, calories - 714*

## INGREDIENTS

- 2 tbsp butter
- 6 pork chops
- 900g cauliflower
- 200g cream cheese
- 160ml double cream
- 230g grated cheddar cheese
- 8g chopped leeks
- 1 clove of garlic, chopped
- Salt and pepper for seasoning

## METHOD

1. Preheat the oven to 200C
2. Take the cauliflower and break it up into small florets
3. Take a pan of boiling water and boil the cauliflower until soft
4. Drain the cauliflower and leave to one side
5. Take a mixing bowl and combine the cream, cream cheese, and three quarters of the grated cheese
6. Add the leaks and combine once more
7. Add the cauliflower to the mixture and combine once more
8. Add the garlic and season, combining once more
9. Transfer the mixture to a baking dish (pre-greased) and sprinkle the rest of the cheese over the top
10. Cook in the oven for half an hour
11. Meanwhile, take a large frying pan and cook the pork chops to your liking
12. Season and serve the chops with the gratin on the side

# VEGETABLE & STEAK KEBABS

*Servings - 2*
*Carbs - 14g, fat - 61g, protein - 55g, calories - 836*

## INGREDIENTS

### For the kebabs:

- 450g sirloin steak
- 1 red onion
- 1 green pepper
- 230g mushrooms
- 4 wooden skewers (metal would also work)

### For the marinade:

- 1 tbsp cider vinegar
- 120ml olive oil
- 3 chopped garlic cloves
- 1 tbsp grated ginger
- 60ml soy sauce
- 0.5 tsp salt
- 0.5 tsp pepper

### For the serving sauce:

- 2 minced garlic cloves
- 1 tsp soy sauce
- 4 tbsp mayonnaise
- 0.5 tsp grated ginger

# METHOD

1. Preheat your grill to 180C
2. Take a mixing bowl and add the cider vinegar, olive oil, 1 tbsp grated ginger, 60ml soy sauce, salt, pepper, and the 3 chopped garlic cloves), combining well
3. Remove 2 tablespoons of the marinade and place in a small bowl
4. Cut the steak up into smaller cubes, around 2 inches in diameter
5. Add the steak to the marinade bowl and ensure it is well coated
6. Allow to marinate for 10 minutes
7. Chop the green pepper and cut the onion into quarter chunks
8. Cut the mushrooms into halves
9. Take your skewers and add the mushrooms, meat, pepper, and onions alternatively
10. Drizzle the rest of the marinade over the kebabs
11. Place the kebabs on the grill and cook for 20 minutes, turning every 5 minutes
12. As you turn the kebabs, brush with a little more marinade from the bowl you set to one side
13. Take a mixing bowl and combine the soy sauce, mayonnaise, grated inner and minced garlic cloves to create a dipping sauce
14. Serve the kebabs with the dipping sauce

# CHICKEN & CASHEW STIR FRY

*Servings - 6*
*Carbs - 8g, fat - 12g, protein - 13g, calories - 199*

## INGREDIENTS

- 230g chicken breasts, cut into cubes
- 2 tbsp sesame oil
- 2 tbsp soy sauce
- 0.5 tsp ground ginger
- 1 tsp sriracha sauce
- 1 tbsp rice vinegar
- 1 red pepper, cut into large pieces
- 110g broccoli florets
- 1 courgette, cut into small pieces
- 2 minced garlic cloves
- 70g cashew nuts, roasted
- 1 tbsp sesame seeds
- 2 sliced spring onions
- Salt and pepper for seasoning

## METHOD

1. Take the chicken chunks and season with ginger, salt and pepper
2. Take a large frying pan and add half of the sesame oil over a medium heat
3. Cook the chicken until brown and cooked all the way through
4. Add the rest of the sesame oil to the pan along with the sriracha, soy sauce, vinegar, courgette, garlic, broccoli, peppers, and mushrooms, combining well
5. Cook for another 10 minutes
6. Add the roasted cashews and cook for another 5 minutes
7. Serve with the chopped spring onions and sesame seeds as a garnish

# CHEESEBURGER IN A CASSEROLE

*Servings - 4*
*Carbs - 11g, fat - 60g, protein - 39g, calories - 749*

## INGREDIENTS

- 2 tbsp butter
- 2 tbsp olive oil
- 450g ground beef
- 1 chopped onion
- 1 cauliflower, cut into florets
- 2 minced garlic cloves
- 1 can of whole tomatoes, fluid drained away
- 2 tbsp tomato paste
- 230g grated cheddar cheese
- 1 tbsp Dijon mustard
- Salt and pepper for seasoning

## METHOD

1. Preheat your oven to 200C
2. Take a baking dish, around 22x30cm size, and grease with a little butter
3. Take a saucepan and boil the cauliflower in salted water until tender
4. Drain the cauliflower and set to one side
5. Take a large frying pan and add the olive oil over a medium heat
6. Add the garlic and onion, cooking until soft
7. Season and add the beef, combining and cook until done throughout
8. Reduce the heat a little and add the tomatoes, tomato paste, cauliflower, mustard, and seasoning, combining well
9. Add three quarters of the cheese and stir until it has melted
10. Transfer the mixture into the baking dish and sprinkle the rest of the cheese over the top
11. Place in the oven and cook for 20 minutes

# CREAMY SHRIMP CASSEROLE

*Servings - 4*
*Carbs - 9g, fat - 50g, protein - 46g, calories - 682*

## INGREDIENTS

- 40g grated parmesan cheese
- 650g white fish of your choice
- 300ml sour cream
- 1 tsp chilli flakes
- 1 tsp saffron
- 3 tbsp olive oil, plus an extra 4 tbsp for the broccoli mash
- 120ml chopped coriander
- 1 minced garlic clove
- 140g peeled shrimp
- 450g broccoli
- Salt and pepper for seasoning

# METHOD

1. Preheat the oven to 200C
2. Take a bang Doha and add the fish inside
3. Season and sprinkle the parmesan over the top
4. Take a medium saucepan and add the sour cream, chilli powder and saffron's combining well
5. Bring to the boil and then turn down to a summer
6. Pour the mixture over the top of the fish, coating well
7. Place in the oven for 20 minutes, ensuring the fish is cooked all the way through
8. Meanwhile, take a large bowl and add the coriander, garlic and 3 tbsp olive oil. Use a hand mixer to combine well
9. Take another large bowl and add the shrimp with the dressing you've just made, combining well
10. Take a saucepan and cook the broccoli in water, until soft
11. Drain the broccoli once cooked and add the rest of the olive oil, with a little salt and pepper
12. Use a hand mixer to create a smooth mash
13. Serve the fish and shrimps with the mash on the side

# BEEF STROGANOFF

*Servings - 4*
*Carbs - 11g, fat - 63g, protein - 40g, calories - 770*

## INGREDIENTS

- 3 tbsp butter
- 2 tbsp olive oil
- 450g ground beef
- 230g crumbled blue cheese
- 350ml sour cream
- 1 chopped onion
- 230g sliced mushrooms
- 1 tbsp thyme (dried)
- 2 courgettes
- Salt and pepper for seasoning

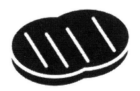

# METHOD

1. Take a large frying pan and add the butter over a medium heat
2. Add the onions and cook until softened
3. Add the beef and cook for another 5 minutes, until browned
4. Add the mushrooms, thyme and season, combining well
5. Cook for another 5 minutes
6. Add the sour cream, blue cheese, and combing
7. Turn the heat up a little and bring the pan's contents to a boil
8. Turn the heat down and allow to simmer for 10 minutes, covered over and stirring every so often
9. Meanwhile, take your courgettes and cut the ends off, slicing in half down the middle
10. Scoop the seeds out of the courgette and use a peeler to create very thin noodles
11. Take a large pan of hot, salted water and bring to the boil
12. Add the courgette "noodles" and cook for a minute
13. Drain and then arrange them on your serving plates
14. Add the olive oil and season a little, tossing the "noodles" until completely covered
15. Serve with the stroganoff on top

# CHEESE & MUSHROOM STUFFED CHICKEN

*Servings - 4*
*Carbs - 9g, fat - 39g, protein - 71g, calories - 690*

## INGREDIENTS

- 4 tbsp olive oil
- 4 chicken breasts
- 1 tbsp soy sauce
- 70g sliced mushrooms
- 1 tbsp fresh thyme leaves
- 200g ricotta cheese
- 1 tsp onion powder
- 4 sprigs fresh thyme
- 28g grated parmesan
- Salt and pepper for seasoning

# METHOD

1. Preheat your oven to 180C
2. Take a large baking tray and line with parchment paper
3. Take your chicken breasts and cut a slit in the sides to create a pocket
4. Use a quarter of the olive oil to rub the outsides of the chicken breasts
5. Season and ensure it is well coated on all sides
6. Take a large frying pan and add another quarter of the olive oil, over a medium heat
7. Add the mushrooms to the pan and cook until crispy, for around 5 minutes
8. Turn the heat down and add the soy sauce and thyme leaves, combining well and cooking for another 3 minutes
9. Take a mixing bowl and add the parmesan, onion powder, ricotta cheese, and a little seasoning
10. Stuff the chicken breasts with the ricotta mixture, ensuring you use equal amounts in all pieces
11. Add a sprig of the thyme on top of each chicken breast
12. Take a frying pan and add the rest of the olive oil, over a medium heat
13. Cook the chicken for 5 minutes on both sides and then transfer to the baking tray
14. Place in the oven for 20 minutes
15. Remove the chicken and cover with foil, allowing it to rest for 10 minutes before serving

# VENISON STEW

*Servings - 6*
*Carbs - 11g, fat - 47g, protein - 32g, calories - 598*

## INGREDIENTS

- 110g butter, plus an extra 2 tbsp butter for the stew
- 1 tsp paprika, plus an extra 1 tsp for the meat
- 60ml olive oil
- 800g venison, cut into chunks of around 1" in size
- 240ml double cream
- 120ml water
- 1 chopped onion
- 1 sliced carrot
- 1 tbsp soy sauce
- 1 minced garlic clove
- 1 tbsp dried rosemary
- 600g cubed celery root
- 3 juniper berries (dried)
- Salt and pepper for seasoning

# METHOD

1. First, create the paprika butter. Take a medium mixing bowl and combine the 110g butter and the 1 tsp paprika to create a smooth paste. Set to one side
2. Take a large frying pan and add half of the olive oil over a medium heat
3. Cook the venison until seared on all sides
4. Season well and add the garlic, onions and carrot, combing again
5. Cook for 2 minutes
6. Add the double cream, water, soy sauce and the spices, combining well
7. Bring the pan to the boil, before adding the gate lid and reducing the heat to low, swimming for up to 1.5 hours. You will need to stir every so often
8. Take a small frying pan and cook the celery root in the rest of the butter, until it's golden brown
9. When your stew has just 20 minutes left to cook, add the celery root and combing
10. Serve the stew in bowls, with the paprika butter over the top

# BAKED FISH WITH VEGETABLES

*Servings - 4*
*Carbs - 14g, fat - 63g, protein - 47g, calories - 857*

## INGREDIENTS

- 90ml olive oil
- 900g white fish fillets, whichever you prefer
- 1 quartered onion
- Half a sliced leek
- 2 chopped red bell peppers
- 2 sliced garlic cloves
- 1 sliced fennel
- 12 cherry tomatoes
- 1 sliced carrot
- 120ml white wine
- 70g pitted olives
- 1 sliced lime
- 1 tbsp fresh parsley
- Salt and pepper for seasoning
- 180ml mayonnaise
- 1 minced garlic clove

# METHOD

1. Preheat your oven to 200C
2. Take a large baking tray and line with parchment paper
3. Cut the fish into pieces and add onto the tray
4. Add the olives, slices of lime, leek, onion, peppers, fennel, tomatoes, and carrot around the fish, in one even layer
5. Add the parsley, 2 sliced garlic cloves, and seasoning
6. Carefully drizzle the white wine over the tray and then drizzle with the oil
7. Make sure the edges of the tray are folded over so the liquids don't escape
8. Place in the oven for 40 minutes
9. Meanwhile, take a small bowl and make the aioli. Add the mayonnaise and the one minced garlic clove with a little seasoning, combining well
10. Serve the fish and vegetables with the aioli on top

# GOULASH WITH BUTTERY CABBAGE

*Servings - 8*
*Carbs - 15g, fat - 42g, protein - 26g, calories - 550*

## INGREDIENTS

- 900g sirloin steak, cubed
- 110g butter, plus an extra 110g for the cabbage
- 180ml water
- 2 onions
- 2 red peppers
- 230g celery root
- 1 tbsp tomato paste
- 1.5 cans of crushed tomatoes
- 2 minced garlic cloves
- 1 tbsp oregano (dried)
- 1 tbsp paprika
- 1 tsp onion powder
- 1 tsp cayenne pepper
- 1 tbsp caraway seeds
- Salt and pepper for seasoning
- 900g shredded cabbage

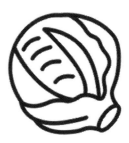

# METHOD

1. Cut the celery, peppers, and onions into pieces of around 1.5cm in length
2. Take a large frying pan and add 55g of the butter over a medium heat
3. Add the onions, peppers, and celery to the pan and cook until soft and golden brown
4. Add the garlic and combine
5. Take a large pan and add the tomatoes, tomato paste, water, and the oregano, paprika, onion powder, cayenne, caraway seeds, and a little salt and pepper, combining well
6. Lower the heat and allow to simmer
7. Meanwhile, take another frying pan and add another 55g of butter. Fry the meat until it is down on all sides
8. Add the meat to the other pan and combine well
9. Allow the pan to simmer for around 2 hours on a low heat. Be sure to stir every so often and if necessary, you can add a little more water
10. Just before serving, season to your liking
11. Before serving, take a frying pan and add the rest of the butter over a medium heat
12. Fry the cabbage and serve with the goulash

# Dessert Recipes

# CLASSIC CINNAMON ROLLS

*Servings - 12*
*Carbs - 1g, fat - 17g, protein - 6g, calories - 183*

## INGREDIENTS

### For the rolls:

- 110g almond flour
- 1 tsp coconut flour
- 32g powdered erythritol
- 2 tbsp cream cheese

- 170g grated mozzarella cheese
- 1 egg
- 0.5 tsp baking powder
- 1 tsp white wine vinegar

### For the roll filling:

- 1 tbsp ground cinnamon
- 32g powdered erythritol

- 110g softened butter

### For the glaze:

- 1.5 tbsp water
- 32g powdered erythritol

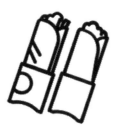

# METHOD

1. Preheat your oven to 185C
2. Melt the cream cheese and mozzarella in a pan over low heat or use a microwave to do the same job
3. Add the almond flour, coconut flour, 32g powdered erythritol, egg, baking powder and white wine vinegar and combine well to create a dough
4. Take a piece of parchment paper and transfer the dough on top. Add another piece of parchment paper on top and use a rolling pin to roll out to a 30x26cm square, around 3mm in thickness
5. Once rolled, discard the top piece of parchment paper
6. Take a mixing bowl and add the filling ingredients - the softened butter, 32g powdered erythritol and the ground cinnamon, combining well
7. Use a spatula to spread the filling over the top of the dough square
8. Carefully roll the dough up tightly, using the parchment paper to move it along
9. Place the dough in the refrigerator for 20 minutes
10. Use a knife to cut the dough into 12 evenly sized pieces
11. Take a large ovenproof baking dish that you can easily place all the rolls inside and line with parchment paper
12. Arrange the rolls inside the baking dish and place in the oven for 12 minutes
13. Remove from the oven and allow to cool
14. Take a medium mixing bowl and mix together the water and remaining powdered erythritol to create the glaze
15. Once the rolls are cool, drizzle the glaze over the top and allow to set before serving

# GINGERBREAD COOKIES

*Servings - 30*
*Carbs - 1g, fat - 6g, protein - 1g, calories - 63*

## INGREDIENTS

- 140g almond flour
- 50g coconut flour
- 160g erythritol
- 1 tbsp ground psyllium husk
- 110g butter
- 3 tsp ground cinnamon
- 2 tsp ground cloves
- 2 tsp ground ginger
- 120ml water
- 1 egg white
- 1 tsp baking powder

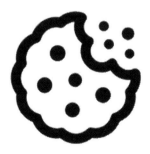

# METHOD

1. Take a medium saucepan and add the cinnamon, cloves, ginger and water together, combining and bringing to the boil over a medium heat
2. Once combined, remove from the heat and add the butter, combining until smooth
3. Take a mixing bowl and combine the almond flour, coconut flour, erythritol, psyllium husk and the baking powder
4. Slowly add the contents of the saucepan to the dry ingredients along with the egg white
5. Combine until the mixture turns into a dough
6. Cover the bowl with plastic wrap and leave in the refrigerator overnight
7. Preheat your oven to 150C
8. Cut the dough ball in half and roll out flat, around 3mm in thickness
9. Use cookie cutters to cut out gingerbread shapes
10. Take a baking sheet and line with parchment paper
11. Transfer the cookies into the baking sheet with a spatula to carefully lift them
12. Place in the oven for 8 minutes, until browned
13. Turn the heat down to 100C and cook for another half an hour until crispy, or a little less if you like them slightly less crunchy
14. Allow to cool before either decorating or simply eating as they are

# CREAMY LOW CARB CHEESECAKE

*Servings - 8*
*Carbs - 16g, fat - 38g, protein - 7g, calories - 388*

## INGREDIENTS

- 110g melted butter
- 230g almond flour
- 55g erythritol for the crust and an extra 110g for the filling
- Pinch of salt
- 900g cream cheese
- 240ml double cream
- The juice and zest of a lemon
- 2 tsp vanilla extract

## METHOD

1. Take a mixing bowl and add the almond flour, 55g erythritol, salt and the melted butter to create a crust mixture

2. Take a springform pan, around 23cm in size and press the crust into the bottom and up the sides

3. Place the pan inside the refrigerator to chill

4. Take a mixing bowl and add the 110g erythritol, cream cheese, lemon zest and juice, double cream and vanilla, combining well until you get a fluffy and smooth mixture

5. Remove the pan from the refrigerator and spread the mixture over the crust evenly

6. Cover the pan with plastic wrap and return to the refrigerator. You should leave the cheesecake preferably overnight, but for three hours at least

# LOW CARB TRES LECHES

*Servings - 8*
*Carbs - 2g, fat - 22g, protein - 6g, calories - 235*

## INGREDIENTS

- 110g almond flour
- 1 tbsp coconut flour
- 1 tsp baking powder
- 110g erythritol
- 3 eggs
- 0.5 tsp lemon juice
- A little butter for greasing
- 120ml double cream, plus an extra 120ml for the cream
- 120ml almond milk
- 1 tbsp vanilla extract
- 2.5 tbsp powdered erythritol, plus an extra 2 tsp for the cream
- 0.25 tsp xanthan gum
- 1 tsp cream cheese

# METHOD

1. Take a large mixing bowl and combine the almond flour, coconut flour, baking powder, erythritol, lemon juice and eggs to create a smooth batter
2. Take a microwavable baking dish around 16x21cm in size and grease with butter
3. Transfer the batter into the dish and smooth over to create a flat layer
4. Place the dish in the microwave and cook for 3.5 minutes on a medium to high heat
5. The cake is cooked when it is firm in the centre; if it isn't firm after 2.5 minutes, cook for another 20 seconds and repeat until cooked
6. Place the cake to one side to cool
7. Meanwhile, take a mixing bowl and combine the 120ml double cream, almond milk, vanilla, 2.5 tbsp powdered erythritol and the xanthan gum
8. Keep stirring the mixture until everything has dissolved and place to one side
9. Take your cooled cake and use a fork to stab holes over the top
10. Pour the mixture over the top of the cake and place in the refrigerator for 2 hours, or preferably until the next day
11. When you're ready to serve, take a hand mixer and beat the cream, powdered erythritol and cream cheese until smooth and stiff
12. Arrange the cream over the top of the cake and serve

# FRUITY RHUBARB TART

*Servings - 8*
*Carbs - 3g, fat - 49g, protein - 11g, calories - 509*

## INGREDIENTS

- 170g almond flour, plus an extra 200g for the filling
- 70g erythritol, plus an extra 110g for the filling
- 85g butter for the crust
- 120g softened butter for the filling
- 200g rhubarb
- 1 tsp vanilla extract
- 21g shredded coconut
- 3 eggs

# METHOD

1. Preheat your oven to 180C
2. Take a tart tin, around 9" in size and grease with little butter
3. Take a mixing bowl and combine the 170g almond flour, coconut and 70g erythritol
4. Melt the 85g butter either over a low heat on the hob or in the microwave
5. Add the melted butter into the mixing bowl and combine well until a dough is created
6. Transfer the dough to the tart tin and press down and around the edges to create a crust
7. Place the tin in the oven for 10 minutes
8. Meanwhile take a stand mixer and add the softened butter and the erythritol inside, beating until a fluffy consistency is achieved
9. Add the eggs, vanilla and almond flour in separate batches and keep beating until smooth
10. Once the tart is cooked, remove from the oven and place to one side to cool, whilst keeping the oven on
11. Peel the rhubarb into strips; you'll need 20 strips in total
12. Use a spoon to add the smooth mixture into the tart base and smooth over
13. Add the rhubarb on top in swirls and push down so they go into the mixture
14. Place back in the oven for 30 minutes and allow to cool before serving

# CHOCOLATE DRIZZLED DOUGHNUTS

*Servings - 8*
*Carbs - 1g, fat - 29g, protein - 7g, calories - 295*

## INGREDIENTS

- 6 eggs
- 50g coconut flour
- 110g erythritol
- 120ml coconut oil
- 0.25 tsp salt
- 025 tsp baking powder
- 1 tsp vanilla
- 0.25 tsp almond extract
- 60ml melted butter, plus an extra 3 tbsp for the drizzle
- 32g powdered erythritol, plus an extra 2 tbsp for the drizzle
- 60g softened cream cheese
- 1 tbsp cocoa powder

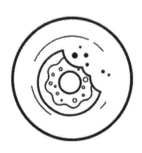

# METHOD

1. Preheat the oven to 175C
2. Take a mixing bowl and add the eggs, coconut flour, erythritol, coconut oil, salt, vanilla almond extract, and baking powder, combining well
3. Take a doughnut pan and transfer the batter inside, filling three quarters of the way up
4. Place in the oven for 20 minutes, until cooked through
5. Take a mixing bowl and add the 60ml melted butter, 32g powdered erythritol, and cream cheese, combining until smooth
6. Once the doughnuts are cool, drip them in the frosting mixture and set aside to rest
7. Meanwhile, make the drizzle by taking a bowl and adding the remaining powdered erythritol, butter and cocoa powder. Combine together until smooth
8. Drizzle over the top of the doughnuts and place in the refrigerator for an hour to set

# CARAMEL & COOKIE SANDWICHES

*Servings - 12*
*Carbs - 1g, fat - 29g, protein - 4g, calories - 284*

## INGREDIENTS

- 70g erythritol plus an extra 110g for the caramel mixture
- 240ml softened butter
- 1 tsp vanilla
- 230g almond flour
- 2 tbsp butter
- 80ml double cream

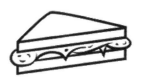

# METHOD

1. Take a large mixing bowl and add the 70g erythritol and softened butter until a smooth consistency is achieved
2. Add the vanilla and combine once more
3. Add the almond flour and continue to combine until smooth
4. Take a piece of parchment paper and transfer the dough on top
5. Roll the parchment paper to create a log shape out of the dough
6. Wrap the parchment around the dough and place in the refrigerator for an hour
7. Meanwhile, take a saucepan over a medium heat and melt the butter
8. Add the rest of the erythritol and the cream and allow simmer
9. Reduce the heat and keep stirring every so often until everything is smooth and the mixture has thickened
10. Remove the pan from the heat and place the contents in a jar to cool
11. Preheat your oven to 160C and line a baking tray with parchment paper
12. Cut the dough into quarter inch thick circles and transfer them to the baking tray
13. Place in the oven for 15 minutes until brown
14. Allow to cool
15. Once the cookies are cool, add some of the caramel mixture on top and then press another cookie round on top, creating a sandwich
16. Repeat with the rest of the cookies

# MINTY MOCHA ICE CREAM

*Servings - 6*
*Carbs - 4g, fat - 38g, protein - 6g, calories - 392*

## INGREDIENTS

- 85g powdered erythritol
- 475ml double cream
- 6 egg yolks
- 55g chopped dark chocolate
- 2 tsp vanilla extract
- 2 tbsp coffee powder
- 0.25 tsp peppermint extract (food grade)
- A pinch of salt

## METHOD

1. Take a large saucepan and add the cream, warming over medium heat and stirring with a whisk
2. Add the dark chocolate and keep whisking as you do so
3. Add the yolks and whisk more
4. Add the coffee powder and erythritol and continue to whisk until everything is well combined
5. Keep whisking until the mixture thickens; this should take around 10 minutes
6. Add the salt, vanilla, and peppermint and combine, tasting to check whether it ends more sweetener or not
7. Place in the refrigerator for an hour
8. Take an ice cream maker and place the mixture inside, following the directions to create your perfect ice cream consistency

# NUTTY FAT BOMBS

*Servings - 4*
*Carbs - 2g, fat - 16g, protein - 2g, calories - 167*

## INGREDIENTS

- 1 tbsp coconut oil
- 38g sugar-free dark chocolate chips
- 45g macadamia nuts, cut into halves
- A pinch of salt

## METHOD

1. Take a mini muffin pan and place three of the macadamia inside
2. Take a microwaveable dish and melt the chocolate chips
3. Add the coconut oil and a little salt, stirring until everything is smooth
4. Add a little of the chocolate mixture over the top of each of the muffin pan inserts, ensuring that the nuts inside are completely covered
5. Add a small amount of salt on top of each muffin insert
6. Place in the freezer for at least half an hour before eating

# DECADENT CHAI LATTE

*Servings - 2*
*Carbs - 1g, fat - 14g, protein - 1g, calories - 133*

## INGREDIENTS

- 475ml water
- 80ml double cream
- 1 tbsp chai tea

## METHOD

1. Follow the instructions on the packet to brew the tea
2. Take a small saucepan and add the cream, heating over a medium heat
3. Add the cream to the heat and stir
4. Serve in two cups and enjoy!

# 2 Weeks Low Carb Meal Prep Plan

Now you know just how delicious following a low carb lifestyle can be! However, it's never easy to actually get started when you're changing the way you eat. To help you out, we've come up with a two week-long meal prep plan. By following this plan as closely as possible, you'll not only ensure that you're on the right track but you'll also see just how easy and delicious following this type of lifestyle can be.

If you don't like one particular meal, feel free to mix it up a little but do try and stick to it as much as you can. Below, you'll see that we've used the recipes already outlined throughout the book but as a bonus, you get one new recipe for every one of the 14 days!

You can also add a dessert any day you like, as long as you stick to the low carb options we've shown you throughout the book.

Bon appetit!

# Day 1

*Breakfast - Salmon, Spinach & Eggs (See page 20)*

*Lunch*

## SIMPLE FISH SALAD
*Servings - 2*
*Carbs - 9g, fat - 34g, protein - 39g, calories - 510*

## INGREDIENTS

- 80ml mayonnaise
- 2 tsp lemon juice
- 0.5 tsp Dijon mustard
- 200g chopped Romaine lettuce
- 200g watercress
- 1 sliced red onion
- 1 sliced cucumber
- 10 halved cherry tomatoes
- 29g pitted olives
- 1 can of tuna in water, drained

## METHOD

1. Take two serving bowls and arrange the romaine lettuce in the bottom of each
2. Add the watercress, onion, cucumber, olives, and tomatoes to each bowl
3. Tip the tuna can into a bowl and take a fork. Flake the tuna and divide between both bowls
4. Take a mixing bowl and combine the mayonnaise, Elgin juice and mustard
5. Drizzle the dressing over the salad bowls

*Dinner - Vegetable & Steak Kebabs (See page 51)*

# Day 2

## *Breakfast*

### HEALTHY CHIA PUDDING
*Servings - 1*
*Carbs - 8g, fat - 56g, protein - 9g, calories - 568*

## INGREDIENTS

- 2 tbsp chia seeds
- 1 can of unsweetened coconut milk
- 0.5 tsp vanilla extract

## METHOD

1. Take a medium sized glass bowl and add all the ingredients inside
2. Combine well
3. Cover the bowl with plastic wrap and place in the refrigerator for at least 54 hours, but preferably overnight
4. The pudding is ready when it has thickened

### *Lunch - Mini Ham Quiches (See page 35)*

### *Dinner - Cauliflower Gratin & Pork Chops (See page 50)*

# Day 3

*Breakfast - Onion & Bacon Breakfast Pancake (See page 21)*

*Lunch - Feta Tabbouleh Bowl (See page 37)*

*Dinner*

## SPICY LAMB STEW
*Servings - 6*
*Carbs - 16g, fat - 44g, protein - 33g, calories - 610*

## INGREDIENTS

- 55g butter
- 60ml water
- 900g lamb shoulder, cut into cubes
- 1 lamb bone
- 1 chopped carrot
- 3 chopped onions
- 2 celery stalks
- 2 chopped garlic cloves
- 1 chopped red chilli pepper
- 1 cinnamon stick
- 2 tbsp curry powder
- 2 tsp salt
- 1 can of crushed tomatoes

## METHOD

1. Take a large pot and add all the ingredients, with the lamb bone in the middle
2. Set your oven to 175C and place the pot inside
3. Cook for 2 hours, stirring occasionally to ensure nothing is sticking to the bottom
4. With around 15 minutes left to go, remove the lamb bone
5. Use a spoon to scoop out the marrow and add back into the stew, stirring to combine
6. Discard the bone
7. Season before serving

# Day 4

*Breakfast - Mackerel & Eggs (See page 23)*

*Lunch*

## HALLOUMI & ASPARAGUS SALAD
*Servings - 4*
*Carbs - 8g, fat - 42g, protein - 21g, calories - 502*

# INGREDIENTS

- 1 tbsp olive oil
- 2 tbsp green pesto
- 60ml mayonnaise
- 1 tbsp fresh lemon juice
- 300g halloumi cheese
- 400g asparagus with the ends chopped
- 85g watercress
- 85g baby spinach
- 140g chopped cherry tomatoes
- 140g sliced avocados
- 200g sliced cucumber
- Salt and pepper for seasoning

# METHOD

1.  Take a large saucepan and add with water to halfway up the side, add some salt
2.  Set the heat to high and bring to the boil
3.  Place the asparagus inside the pan and cook for 5 minutes
4.  Drain the asparagus and place to one side
5.  Cut the halloumi into 1cm thick slices
6.  Take a large pan and add the oil over a medium heat
7.  Cook the halloumi for around 3 minutes on each side; it should be crispy before you turn it
8.  Place to one side and keep warm
9.  Take a large serving bowl and add the spinach and watercress, tossing to combine
10. Add the tomatoes, avocado, and cucumber on top
11. Add the asparagus
12. Add the halloumi on top
13. Take a small mixing bowl and mix the pesto and the pesto, mayonnaise and lemon juice together
14. Drizzle over the top of the salad and serve

*Dinner - Chicken & Cashew Stir Fry (See page 53)*

# Day 5

***Breakfast***

**MORNING MUFFINS**

*Servings - 6*
*Carbs - 2g, fat - 26g, protein - 26g, calories - 353*

## INGREDIENTS

- 2 chopped spring onions
- 12 eggs
- 2 tbsp green pesto
- 170g grated cheddar cheese
- 140g cooked bacon
- Salt and pepper for seasoning

## METHOD

1. Preheat your oven to 175C
2. Take a muffin tin and grease the insides with butter
3. Place the cooked bacon and chopped spring onion into the bottom of each muffin insert
4. Take a bowl and combine the pesto, eggs, and seasoning until smooth
5. Divide the mixture between each muffin insert
6. Sprinkle the cheddar cheese on top of each insert
7. Place in the oven and back for 20 minutes, until golden brown

***Lunch - Shrimp & Cabbage Stir Fry (See page 36)***

***Dinner - Cheeseburger in a Casserole (See page 54)***

# Day 6

*Breakfast - Turkey & Mustard Breakfast Sandwich (See page 22)*

## Lunch

### CHEESY MEATBALLS

*Servings - 4*
*Carbs - 5g, fat - 49g, protein - 39g, calories - 628*

# INGREDIENTS

- 450g ground beef
- 3 tbsp olive oil
- 1 egg
- 60g grated Parmesan cheese
- 140g fresh mozzarella cheese, torn into pieces
- 1 can of whole tomatoes
- 55g butter
- 0.5 tbsp dried basil
- 1 tsp garlic powder
- 0.5 tsp onion powder
- 0.5 tsp black pepper
- 1 tsp salt
- 2 tbsp chopped parsley
- 200g fresh spinach

# METHOD

1. Take a large mixing bowl and add the beef, parmesan cheese, salt, egg, garlic powder, onion powder, black pepper and combine well
2. Use your hands to create meatballs, around 30g in weight each
3. Take a large frying pan and add the oil over a medium heat
4. Cook the meatballs, turning regularly to ensure they brown evenly
5. Once browned, turn down the heat a little and add the can of tomatoes, simmering for 15 minutes
6. Season to your liking and add the parsley, combining again
7. Take another frying pan and add the butter
8. Add the spinach and cook for 2 minutes, stirring all the time
9. Season and add the spinach to the main pain
10. Serve the meatballs with the mozzarella cheese on top

*Dinner - Creamy Shrimp Casserole (See page 55)*

# Day 7

*Breakfast - Bacon & Avocado Eggs (See page 24)*

*Lunch - Low Carb Tuna Burgers (See page 38)*

*Dinner*

## SPICY MEXICAN CASSEROLE
*Servings - 4*
*Carbs - 8g, fat - 66g, protein - 50g, calories - 840*

## INGREDIENTS

- 85g butter
- 650g ground beef
- 1 can of crushed tomatoes
- 230g grated cheddar cheese
- 55g pickled jalapeño peppers, chopped
- 3 tbsp Tex-Mex seasoning/taco or fajita seasoning

## METHOD

1. Preheat your oven to 200C
2. Take a large frying pan and add the butter over a medium heat
3. Add the beef and cook until browned
4. Add the tomatoes and the Tex-Mex seasoning, combining well
5. Allow the mixture to simmer for 5 minutes
6. Take a baking dish around 23cm in size and grease with little butter
7. Transfer the mixture to the baking dish
8. Add the cheese and jalapeños over the top in an even layer
9. Place in the oven for 20 minutes, until bubbling and golden brown

# Day 8

*Breakfast*

## FETA & CHORIZO EGG POTS

*Servings - 1*
*Carbs - 7g, fat - 37g, protein - 28g, calories - 474*

## INGREDIENTS

- 1 tsp olive oil
- 2 eggs
- 55g spinach, fresh works best but frozen is also fine
- 55g chorizo
- 55g halved cherry tomatoes
- 60ml crumbled feta cheese
- Salt and pepper for seasoning

## METHOD

1. Preheat your oven to 200C
2. Take two regular sized ramekin dish and grease with little olive oil
3. Crack one egg into each ramekin
4. Add the chorizo evenly between the two ramekins, along with the tomatoes and the crumbled feta cheese
5. Place the ramekins in the oven and cook for 12 minutes
6. Season and serve

*Lunch - Mozzarella Beef Salad (See page 39)*

*Dinner - Baked Fish With Vegetables (See page 63)*

# Day 9

***Breakfast - Morning Caprese Omelette (See page 28)***

***Lunch***

## MEDITERRANEAN PLATE
*Servings - 1*
*Carbs - 7g, fat - 41g, protein - 27g, calories - 516*

# INGREDIENTS

- 1 tbsp olive oil
- 85g prosciutto
- 1 boiled egg, sliced
- 1 tsp fresh lemon juice
- 28g crumbled feta cheese
- 2 halved cherry tomatoes
- 14g leafy greens, mixed
- 55g sliced avocado
- 14g sliced spring onion
- Salt and pepper for seasoning

# METHOD

1. Lay the leafy greens out on your serving plate
2. Arrange the prosciutto on top, followed by the sliced avocado, spring onions, cherry tomatoes, and the sliced boiled egg
3. Sprinkle the feta cheese over the top
4. Take a mixing bowl and combine the olive oil and lemon juice
5. Drizzle the dressing over the plate and season with salt and pepper for serving

***Dinner - Beef Stroganoff (See page 57)***

# Day 10

*Breakfast - Avocado & Swede Fritters (See page 26)*

*Lunch - Leek & Broccoli Soup With Cheesy Chips (See page 41)*

*Dinner*

## CHILI WITHOUT THE BEANS
*Servings - 4*
*Carbs - 8g, fat - 59g, protein - 50g, calories - 779*

## INGREDIENTS

- 800g ground beef
- 3 tbsp olive oil
- 240ml beef broth
- 1 diced tomato
- 2 sliced jalapeños
- 2 tsp smoked paprika powder
- 2 tbsp chilli powder
- 2 tsp cumin
- 2 tbsp tomato paste
- 2 chopped garlic cloves
- Salt and pepper to taste

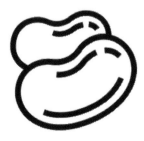

# METHOD

1. Take a large stock pot and add the oil over a medium heat
2. Add the garlic and onion and fry for a couple of minutes, until soft
3. Add the smoked paprika powder, chilli powder, and the cumin, stirring to combine
4. Add the ground beef and cook until browned
5. Add the tomato paste, tomato, broth and the jalapeños and combine
6. Bring the pot to the boil and then reduce the heat to a simmer for 10 minutes
7. Keep stirring every so often and season to your taste

# Day 11

*Breakfast - Avocado Eggs Benedict (See page 32)*

*Lunch*

## GARLICKY SHRIMPS
*Servings - 4*
*Carbs - 6g, fat - 12g, protein - 34g, calories - 280*

## INGREDIENTS

- 900g shrimp, deveined and peeled
- 2 tbsp olive oil
- 2 tbsp sesame seeds
- 2 chopped garlic cloves
- 230g sliced bok choy
- 4 sliced spring onions
- 1 sliced red bell pepper
- 2 tbsp soy sauce

## METHOD

1. Take a large frying pan and add half of the oil over a medium heat
2. Add the garlic and sesame seeds, along with the shrimp and cook for 2 minutes,
3. Add the rest of the oil, along with the soy sauce and the bok choy, and red bell pepper, combining well
4. Cook for 5 minutes, until everything is tender
5. Transfer to serving bowls with the spring onions sprinkled over the top

*Dinner - Cheese & Mushroom Stuffed Chicken (See page 59)*

# Day 12

*Breakfast*

## LETTUCE BREAKFAST WRAPS
*Servings - 2*
*Carbs - 4g, fat - 53g, protein - 31g, calories - 631*

## INGREDIENTS

- 3 tbsp mayonnaise
- 55g lettuce
- Half an avocado, pitted and peeled
- 1 sliced tomato
- 170g sliced bacon
- Salt and pepper for seasoning

## METHOD

1. Take a large frying pan over a medium heat
2. Add the bacon and cook for around 5 minutes
3. Once cooked, remove from the pan and place on paper towels
4. Cut each slice of bacon in half
5. Arrange your lettuce leaves on the serving plates
6. Add a little mayonnaise on top of each leaf
7. Add a slice of tomato on top of each leaf
8. Add 3 slices of bacon on top of each leaf
9. Top with a slice of avocado and season

*Lunch - Traditional Gumbalaya (See page 43)*

*Dinner - Venison Stew (See page 61)*

# Day 13

*Breakfast - Breakfast Taco turnover (See page 29)*

*Lunch - Cauliflower & Mushroom Risotto (See page 45)*

*Dinner*

## KALE & CHICKEN SOUP

*Servings - 6*
*Carbs - 9g, fat - 31g, protein - 32g, calories - 447*

## INGREDIENTS

- 450g shredded cooked chicken
- 3 tbsp olive oil
- 950ml chicken broth
- 280g kale
- 450g chopped cauliflower
- 50g minced ginger
- 2 chopped garlic cloves
- 280g cream cheese
- 2 chopped onions
- Salt and pepper for seasoning

# METHOD

1. Take a large soup pot and add the oil over a medium heat
2. Add the garlic, onion, ginger, and cauliflower and cook for 2 minutes
3. Add the cream cheese and season, combining well
4. Turn the heat down and stir until the cream cheese has melted
5. Add the kale and broth, combining well
6. Use a food processor to create a smooth mixture
7. Turn the heat up to high and allow to boil, before turning down to a simmer for 10 more minutes
8. Add the chicken and combine
9. Season before serving

# Day 14

***Breakfast - Berry Breakfast Smoothie (See page 31)***

## *Lunch*

### STUFFED CABBAGE PARCELS IN GRAVY
*Servings - 4*
*Carbs - 11g, fat - 75g, protein - 38g, calories - 866*

## INGREDIENTS

- 450g whole leaves of savoy cabbage
- 55g butter
- 200g shredded cauliflower
- 1 chopped onion
- 160ml double cream, plus an extra 240ml for the gravy
- 650g ground beef
- 1 tbsp soy sauce
- Salt and pepper for seasoning

# METHOD

1. Preheat your oven to 200C
2. Fill a saucepan with water and bring to the boil
3. Boil the cabbage leaves for 4 minutes and set aside to drain
4. Take a frying pan and add half the butter over a medium heat
5. Fry the onion and cauliflower and season with salt and pepper
6. Set aside to cool down
7. Take a mixing bowl and add the onion and cauliflower, along with the 160ml cream, ground beef, and seasoning
8. Comb well and add a spoonful of each to each cabbage leaf, right in the centre
9. Fold over each side of the leaf and roll the leaf up
10. Take a frying pan and add the rest of the butter over a medium heat
11. Fry the cabbage parcels on each side for a few minutes, until they grow slightly brown
12. Take an ovenproof dish and grease with a little butter
13. Arrange the cabbage parcels inside and place in the oven for half an hour
14. Take a saucepan and add the rest of the cream and the sauce sac, bringing to the boil
15. Turn the heat down and allow to simmer for 5 minutes. The gravy should thicken
16. Serve the cabbage leaves with the gravy poured over the top - one serving is three parcels per person

*Dinner - Goulash With Buttery Cabbage (See page 65)*

# Conclusion

Now you know exactly how to follow and enjoy the low carb lifestyle, there's no stopping you!

Learning how to cook delicious and healthy meals is a wonderful habit to get into and before long, you'll be impressing your loved ones with your new recipe knowledge!

Of course, the recipes in this book aren't all you can eat on this low carb journey you've decided to embark upon. These recipes are designed to show you how easy the lifestyle can be and to get you started. As you learn, you'll start to adapt your own recipes and create dishes that are not only low in carb amount, but are delicious, wholesome, and extremely filling at the same time.

You've already taken the best first step by choosing to read this book. Hopefully you'll soon start to cook your first recipe, if you haven't already!

All that's left to say is good luck with your new low carb journey and enjoy all the delicious meals you're yet to create.

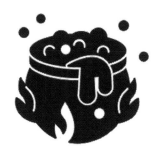

# Disclaimer

This book contains opinions and ideas of the author and is meant to teach the reader informative and helpful knowledge while due care should be taken by the user in the application of the information provided. The instructions and strategies are possibly not right for every reader and there is no guarantee that they work for everyone. Using this book and implementing the information/ recipes therein contained is explicitly your own responsibility and risk. This work with all its contents, does not guarantee correctness, completion, quality or correctness of the provided information. Misinformation or misprints cannot be completely eliminated.

Printed in Great Britain
by Amazon

65299824R00066